My Favorite Smoothie Recipes Book

A record of the best smoothie recipes that I have found or created so far

Journal Easy

© 2014

www.journaleasy.com – making journal writing effortless

Smoothie Name:

Ingredients:

Comments:

Smoothie Name:

Ingredients:

Comments:

Smoothie Name:

Ingredients:

Comments:

Smoothie Name:

Ingredients:

Comments:

Smoothie Name:

Ingredients:

Comments:

Smoothie Name:

Ingredients:

Comments:

Smoothie Name:

Ingredients:

Comments:

Smoothie Name:

Ingredients:

Comments:

Smoothie Name:

Ingredients:

Comments:

Smoothie Name:

Ingredients:

Comments:

Smoothie Name:

Ingredients:

Comments:

Smoothie Name:

Ingredients:

Comments:

Smoothie Name:

Ingredients:

Comments:

Smoothie Name:

Ingredients:

Comments:

Smoothie Name:

Ingredients:

Comments:

Smoothie Name:

Ingredients:

Comments:

Smoothie Name:

Ingredients:

Comments:

Smoothie Name:

Ingredients:

Comments:

Smoothie Name:

Ingredients:

Comments:

Smoothie Name:

Ingredients:

Comments:

Smoothie Name:

Ingredients:

Comments:

Smoothie Name:

Ingredients:

Comments:

Smoothie Name:

Ingredients:

Comments:

Smoothie Name:

Ingredients:

Comments:

Smoothie Name:

Ingredients:

Comments:

Smoothie Name:

Ingredients:

Comments:

Smoothie Name:

Ingredients:

Comments:

Smoothie Name:

Ingredients:

Comments:

Smoothie Name:

Ingredients:

Comments:

Smoothie Name:

Ingredients:

Comments:

Smoothie Name:

Ingredients:

Comments:

Smoothie Name:

Ingredients:

Comments:

Smoothie Name:

Ingredients:

Comments:

Smoothie Name:

Ingredients:

Comments:

Smoothie Name:

Ingredients:

Comments:

Smoothie Name:

Ingredients:

Comments:

Smoothie Name:

Ingredients:

Comments:

Smoothie Name:

Ingredients:

Comments:

Smoothie Name:

Ingredients:

Comments:

Smoothie Name:

Ingredients:

Comments:

Smoothie Name:

Ingredients:

Comments:

Smoothie Name:

Ingredients:

Comments:

Smoothie Name:

Ingredients:

Comments:

Smoothie Name:

Ingredients:

Comments:

Smoothie Name:

Ingredients:

Comments:

Smoothie Name:

Ingredients:

Comments:

Smoothie Name:

Ingredients:

Comments:

Smoothie Name:

Ingredients:

Comments:

Smoothie Name:

Ingredients:

Comments:

Smoothie Name:

Ingredients:

Comments:

Smoothie Name:

Ingredients:

Comments:

Smoothie Name:

Ingredients:

Comments:

Smoothie Name:

Ingredients:

Comments:

Smoothie Name:

Ingredients:

Comments:

Smoothie Name:

Ingredients:

Comments:

Smoothie Name:

Ingredients:

Comments:

Smoothie Name:

Ingredients:

Comments:

Smoothie Name:

Ingredients:

Comments:

Smoothie Name:

Ingredients:

Comments:

Smoothie Name:

Ingredients:

Comments:

Smoothie Name:

Ingredients:

Comments:

Smoothie Name:

Ingredients:

Comments:

Smoothie Name:

Ingredients:

Comments:

Smoothie Name:

Ingredients:

Comments:

Smoothie Name:

Ingredients:

Comments:

Smoothie Name:

Ingredients:

Comments:

Smoothie Name:

Ingredients:

Comments:

Smoothie Name:

Ingredients:

Comments:

Smoothie Name:

Ingredients:

Comments:

Smoothie Name:

Ingredients:

Comments:

Smoothie Name:

Ingredients:

Comments:

Smoothie Name:

Ingredients:

Comments:

Smoothie Name:

Ingredients:

Comments:

Smoothie Name:

Ingredients:

Comments:

Smoothie Name:

Ingredients:

Comments:

Smoothie Name:

Ingredients:

Comments:

Smoothie Name:

Ingredients:

Comments:

Smoothie Name:

Ingredients:

Comments:

Smoothie Name:

Ingredients:

Comments:

Smoothie Name:

Ingredients:

Comments:

Smoothie Name:

Ingredients:

Comments:

Smoothie Name:

Ingredients:

Comments:

Smoothie Name:

Ingredients:

Comments:

Smoothie Name:

Ingredients:

Comments:

Smoothie Name:

Ingredients:

Comments:

Smoothie Name:

Ingredients:

Comments:

Smoothie Name:

Ingredients:

Comments:

Smoothie Name:

Ingredients:

Comments:

Smoothie Name:

Ingredients:

Comments:

Smoothie Name:

Ingredients:

Comments:

Smoothie Name:

Ingredients:

Comments:

Smoothie Name:

Ingredients:

Comments:

Smoothie Name:

Ingredients:

Comments:

Smoothie Name:

Ingredients:

Comments:

Smoothie Name:

Ingredients:

Comments:

Smoothie Name:

Ingredients:

Comments:

Smoothie Name:

Ingredients:

Comments:

Smoothie Name:

Ingredients:

Comments:

Smoothie Name:

Ingredients:

Comments:

Smoothie Name:

Ingredients:

Comments:

Smoothie Name:

Ingredients:

Comments:

Smoothie Name:

Ingredients:

Comments:

Smoothie Name:

Ingredients:

Comments:

Smoothie Name:

Ingredients:

Comments:

Smoothie Name:

Ingredients:

Comments:

Smoothie Name:

Ingredients:

Comments:

Smoothie Name:

Ingredients:

Comments:

Smoothie Name:

Ingredients:

Comments:

Smoothie Name:

Ingredients:

Comments:

Smoothie Name:

Ingredients:

Comments:

Smoothie Name:

Ingredients:

Comments:

Smoothie Name:

Ingredients:

Comments:

Smoothie Name:

Ingredients:

Comments:

Smoothie Name:

Ingredients:

Comments:

Smoothie Name:

Ingredients:

Comments:

Smoothie Name:

Ingredients:

Comments:

Smoothie Name:

Ingredients:

Comments:

Smoothie Name:

Ingredients:

Comments:

Smoothie Name:

Ingredients:

Comments:

Smoothie Name:

Ingredients:

Comments:

Smoothie Name:

Ingredients:

Comments:

Smoothie Name:

Ingredients:

Comments:

Smoothie Name:

Ingredients:

Comments:

Smoothie Name:

Ingredients:

Comments:

Smoothie Name:

Ingredients:

Comments:

Smoothie Name:

Ingredients:

Comments:

Smoothie Name:

Ingredients:

Comments:

Smoothie Name:

Ingredients:

Comments:

Smoothie Name:

Ingredients:

Comments:

Smoothie Name:

Ingredients:

Comments:

Smoothie Name:

Ingredients:

Comments:

Smoothie Name:

Ingredients:

Comments:

Smoothie Name:

Ingredients:

Comments:

Smoothie Name:

Ingredients:

Comments:

Smoothie Name:

Ingredients:

Comments:

Smoothie Name:

Ingredients:

Comments:

Smoothie Name:

Ingredients:

Comments:

Smoothie Name:

Ingredients:

Comments:

Smoothie Name:

Ingredients:

Comments:

Smoothie Name:

Ingredients:

Comments:

Smoothie Name:

Ingredients:

Comments:

Smoothie Name:

Ingredients:

Comments:

Smoothie Name:

Ingredients:

Comments:

Smoothie Name:

Ingredients:

Comments:

Smoothie Name:

Ingredients:

Comments:

Smoothie Name:

Ingredients:

Comments:

Smoothie Name:

Ingredients:

Comments:

Smoothie Name:

Ingredients:

Comments:

Smoothie Name:

Ingredients:

Comments:

Smoothie Name:

Ingredients:

Comments:

My Favorite Smoothie Books & Resources

If you don't have a blender or smoothie maker yet, go to: www.vitalityjuicers.com in the USA & Canada or www.vitalityjuicers.co.uk in the UK. These sites research & find the best juicers & blenders that can be bought online.

My Favorite Smoothie Books & Resources

My Favorite Smoothie Books & Resources

My Favorite Smoothie Books & Resources

www.ingramcontent.com/pod-product-compliance
Lightning Source LLC
La Vergne TN
LVHW011710060526
838200LV00051B/2848